7 Day Quick Start to Green Juicing

The Complete Guide to Getting Started Juicing, Why It's Beneficial, Along With a 7 Day Green Juice Plan

By. Mariam Turay

ISBN-13: 978-1489554130

Thank you for your purchase of this book.

For your free bonus Visit
http://www.greenjuiceaday.com/kindle-bonus

Also join our Green Juice A Day community at
http://www.facebook.com/GreenJuiceADay

For additional support on your juicing journey.

Table of Contents

Introduction 3-5

Disclaimer 6

My Story 7-10

Why Juice? 11-14

Juicing vs. Blending 15-16

Why Drink Green Juices? 17-18

Getting Started 19-36

Selecting a Juicer 19

    Types of Juicers 19-22

    Where to Buy Juicers 23

    Other Equipment 24

Selecting Produce 25

Organic vs. Conventional 25-27

How to Buy Affordable Organic Produce 28-30

Fruit and Vegetable Prep for Juicing 31-32

Storing Your Produce 32-34

Storing Your Juices 35

Proper Juicing Etiquette 36

7 Day Juice Plan 37-51

    Monday 38-39

Tuesday 40-41

Wednesday 42-43

Thursday 44-45

Friday 46-47

Saturday 48-49

Sunday 50-51

Shopping List 52

How to a Make Green Juice Template 53-59

Fruit and Vegetable Flavor Families................60-61

Vegetable & Fruit Substitution List 62-65

Frequently Asked Questions 66-69

Conclusion 70

Introduction

The choices that we make today are affecting our health profile, not only today but in years to come, and may be playing a role in what we may die from.

It has always been my belief that our bodies have the ability to heal themselves, so long as we give them what they need. In my experience, this has become a truth. Research is showing that the quality of food you put in your body can either improve your health or cause many of the diseases that are prevalent in this country and worldwide. Diseases such as heart disease, cancer, kidney and liver disease, and diabetes are among the top killers in the United States and of many developed countries. It is of no surprise now that science is proving these diseases are related to diet and nutrition. A poor diet plus a negative lifestyle equals death and disease.

So what sort of foods can improve our health? Real foods. Whole living foods. A diet that incorporates fresh fruits and vegetables. And I'm not referring to a little side salad at dinner. Every meal should have fresh fruits and vegetables, both raw and cooked. I'm not just saying this to say it; organizations like the American Cancer Society and the National Cancer Institute are now recommending at least five servings of fruits and vegetables each day as a means of preventing cancer. There is an undeniable correlation between nutrition and health.

The recommendations are out there, yet many of us don't know how to start incorporating more fruits and vegetables or simply don't have enough time. That's where juicing comes in. Although juicing may seem like the new fad, it has been practiced for quite some time. We can trace juicing back to 300 BC. Hippocrates, known as the father of Western medicine, was an advocate of juicing for treating diseases as well as maintaining health. In the past century many have used juicing to overcome debilitating diseases and improve their health. Jay Kordich (the Juice Man) used juicing and a clean diet to cure himself of bladder cancer. Dr. Max Gerson founder of the Gerson Institute and the Gerson Therapy used juicing as a way to cure himself of horrible migraines and tuberculosis. The Gerson Institute has had great success in curing many people of cancer, heart disease, diabetes and many other chronic diseases through a holistic approach that incorporates green juices. These are a few examples, but there are many out there who can attest to the benefits of juicing.

In this book you will discover why incorporating fresh juices into your daily routine can improve your overall health. Here's what you will learn in this book:

- Why juicing is so beneficial
- The difference between juices and smoothies
- How to juice
- How to find a juicer that's right for you
- How to juice on a budget
- Tips on finding affordable organic produce
- How to store your produce to minimize spoilage
- A chart of the different fruit and vegetable flavors
- A list of fruit and vegetable substitutions
- A simple formula on how to make a green juice for endless combinations
- A 7 day juice a day plan with a shopping list

You should know that my recommendations throughout this book are based on my experience, research, and/or stories shared with me. I hold no endorsements as I write this, no fluff, just pure truth. Please know that I am not a medical doctor. All the information, stories and experiences are for informational purposes only. Please do your own research and consult a licensed medical doctor should you start to make changes in your diet, preferably one that understands the benefits juicing offers to your health.

7 Day Quick Start to Green Juicing

By: Mariam Turay of

http://www.GreenJuiceADay.com

The information contained in this guide is for informational purposes only.

I am not a medical doctor. The information presented is based on experience and/or scientific research. You should always seek the advice of a licensed medical doctor before making any changes to your current diet.

No part of this publication shall be reproduced, transmitted, or sold in whole or in part in any form, without the prior written consent of the author.

Users of this guide are advised to do their own due diligence when it comes to making health decisions and the information and products that have been provided should be independently verified by your own qualified health professionals. By reading this guide, you agree that I am not responsible for any decision you chose to make relating to any information presented in this guide.

My Story

"The doctor of the future will give no medication, but will interest his patients in the care of the human frame, diet and in the cause and prevention of disease." ~ Thomas Edison

Before we get started with juicing, I want to share a little about myself and my juicing journey. I grew up eating foods I thought were healthy. My parents, believing that what was sold at the grocery store was high quality and nutritious, felt that the foods they were feeding me and my brothers was beneficial. We are learning more now that not all foods in the grocery stores are healthy. A lot of the convenience foods sold in markets are either too high in sugar, salt, and/or fat and contain a load of harmful synthetic chemicals, toxins and food dyes that may increase your risk of cancer, diabetes, heart disease, and more. I grew up eating the standard American diet along with some ethnic African cuisines. My favorite foods as a child were fried chicken, eggs, French fries and Wendy's Frosties, and chili. If you asked me then what foods would I want if stuck on a deserted island it would probably be those.

Needless to say as I approached my twenties some problems arose. Even though I was physically active, I was still overweight, tired all the time, and lacked energy, but most importantly suffered from anxiety and depression. If you don't know what it's like to have anxiety attacks let me paint a picture for you. Imagine having this daily feeling like something horrible is going to happen, feeling you're going to die. If you don't know what that feels like, imagine a time you were on an airplane and hit a big pocket of turbulence. For a few seconds your heart stops and you can suddenly feel your stomach in your throat with the feeling the plane may crash. Now imagine having that feeling every day and not being able to control it. This is what I dealt with on a daily basis.

It wasn't until I had a severe attack that I paid a visit to the doctor. I remember this day clearly, because I truly thought I was going to die. I was lying in bed watching TV. All of a sudden I couldn't move. I thought I was paralyzed. I had sharp stabbing pains in my chest and numbness throughout my body. I thought I was having a heart attack at twenty-one years old. That feeling where you can't move or call anyone for help was scary. When I returned from the doctor I was prescribed Percocet, a pain reliever for severe pain. I was taking a strong pain reliever and it was not helping at all. I still felt like I was going to die and had sharp pains in my chest. They ran a couple of tests on me and found there was nothing "physically" wrong nor did I have any heart issues.

Despite what the doctors said, I still felt horrible. To reduce my pain my doctor prescribed tranquilizers. Scary stuff. Tranquillizers work by reducing brain function and slowing down the entire central nervous system. Now does that sound right to you? Instead of fixing the problem they wanted to cover it up. Biology and nutrition were my majors, so I knew a thing or two about the central nervous system (CNS). The CNS makes up our brain and spinal cord. It's responsible for sending, receiving, and interpreting information throughout the body. So the idea of this drug slowing down rubbed me the wrong way. Deep down I just knew there had to be another solution: one that would fix my problems completely so that I wouldn't have to deal with the daily anxiety and frequent attacks.

I stumbled upon raw foods and juicing as I searched for holistic ways to treat my anxiety. I learned about how people used juicing along with clean foods to reverse severe health issues, like diabetes, cancer, obesity, fatigue, insomnia, heart disease, and many other issues people face on a daily basis. Suddenly, a light bulb went off. In order for me to regain my health I needed to return back to nature. For the past twenty years the majority of my diet consisted of food-like products that didn't really nourish my body. My body was lacking in the necessary minerals, vitamins, and nutrients it needed to function optimally. So I purchased as many books as I could obtain, read several dozen blogs, and researched a ton to begin my transformation.

The truth is my transformation was not easy and at times I struggled. You see or read about someone having success through juicing, or whatever it is, and in your brain all you see is the final result, not the steps it took to get there. I underestimated what it would take to get to the end. In fact, I wish there had been more information out there. For instance, it's not best to jump into an extended juice fast if your current diet is not the best and/or you've never done one before or if you're just looking for a quick fix to lose weight. I jumped head first into a 30 day juice fast which took a lot of will power to get through. I went through lots of detoxing and emotional release during that time, which was very difficult while in school. I can't tell you how many epic juice fails I've had. It's best to take things slowly. Don't beat yourself up if you hit bumps in the road. It's the little steps that we make that will lead to a permanent road of success. We don't realize that the road to optimal health is not a sprint, but a marathon. Each of us will end that marathon at different times. Remember, there is no quick fix or magic pill to optimal health. It was a roller coaster of a ride, but I made it through.

Some of the benefits I experienced from incorporating juicing and clean foods into my diet include a 25lb weight loss, more energy, better skin, and better sleep. Most importantly, I am free of the anxiety and depression I once struggled with leading me to an overall sense of happiness. That is why I'm writing this book: to introduce you to juicing and how it can improve your health and also give you everything you need to know to succeed. All it takes is a green juice a day. By incorporating a fresh glass of a green juice a day you will no doubt experience an improvement in your health. Drinking fresh juice will open the door to adopting healthier eating habits, increase your daily requirements of fruits and vegetables, and help you achieve your weight loss goals.

So if you're ready for a new you, turn the page and let's get started.

Why Juice?

Let's face it, Americans are sick, overweight, and have a multitude of health problems. The CDC reports that **more than two-thirds (68.8%) of adults are considered to be overweight or obese.** Over the past 20 years there has been a constant decline in the health of our country. We are eating way more foods than any other country, yet we are undernourished, and lacking necessary nutrients and minerals our body needs to function optimally. Scientists are now acknowledging that a poor diet is a major contributor to many of the diseases prevalent in the United States and many other developed nations. The U.S. Department of Agriculture (USDA) has found that Americans have failed miserably to meet the recommended daily allowances (RDA) of vitamins and minerals. Take for instance potassium. Potassium is a necessary mineral for life, yet **90% of Americans are deficient**. Potassium is necessary for the heart, kidneys, and other organs to function properly, and helps regulate blood pressure. The CDC reports that **1 in 3 Americans have high blood pressure. High blood pressure is a major risk factor for cardiovascular disease, stroke, and kidney disease.** I've only mentioned one mineral; however, you can see how critical vitamins and minerals are to our health. "You can trace every sickness, every disease, and every ailment to a mineral deficiency." – Dr. Linus Pauling (Winner of two Nobel Prizes).

There is a simple solution to this big problem. **The solution is to include a variety of fresh organic fruits and vegetables in your diet daily.** In our fast-paced society we often sacrifice health for what is easiest and quickest. Getting the daily allowances of fruits and vegetables can sometimes be difficult. One of the best ways to fulfill the recommended daily allowances is through **juicing**. Let me first state that juicing is not a cure-all. The point of juicing is to get the maximum amount of vitamins, minerals, enzymes, and phytochemicals directly into your body, so that your body can perform its duties optimally. Before you head out to your local store and pick up a Naked juice or an Odwalla bottle, know that when I say juicing I mean fresh juices that you make yourself or pick up from a juice bar. Products such as Naked and Odwalla are pasteurized (vitamins/minerals are cooked out) and filled with sugar and other chemicals not beneficial to your body. Those sugar-filled "fruit juices" are lacking in life force, vitamins, minerals, antioxidants, and many health properties fresh fruits and vegetable juice provide.

Fresh fruits and vegetables are low in fat and are key sources for essential nutrients. Research consistently shows that **people who consume the greatest quantity of fruits and vegetables are about 50% less likely to develop cancer** as those who eat little fresh fruits and vegetables. Fruits and vegetables hold the key to preventing many modern diseases.

So why juice? There is no health product or supplement on the market that compares to a healthy diet paired with daily juicing. One quart of fresh green juice supplies the nutrition equivalent to approx. five pounds of solid fruits and vegetables. I don't know anyone that can consume that much produce in a day, let alone in one sitting. Besides, who wants to sit there and chew all those fruits and vegetables?

When you process the fruits and vegetables through a juicer, the juicer extracts all the fluids and nutrients from the solids. Fresh juices are quickly digested and assimilated by the body. Fresh juice is digested in as little as 15 minutes, with very little effort or exertion on the digestive system. This means once you consume your fresh juice, the vitamins, minerals, phytochemicals (plant chemical compounds, like resveratrol, a natural cancer killer), and antioxidants are immediately available to your cells and tissues. Solid foods have to be digested over many hours before nourishment becomes available to the cells and tissues of the body. This instant blast of natural nutrient has been shown to boost health, enhance immunity, help prevent cancer and cardiovascular disease, and provide a natural source of energy.

Top 13 Benefits of Juicing

Easy Assimilation: enzymes, phytochemicals, vitamins, and trace minerals are rapidly available for the cells and tissues in the body within 15 minutes.

Extremely Hydrating: our cells consist mainly of water, which is essential to proper cell function, hence the daily recommendations of 8 glasses of water a day; juicing supplies the water you need to replenish lost fluids.

Promotes Alkalinity: vital for proper immune function. Diseases, infections, inflammation, pain, and cancer all thrive in an acidic environment.

Cleansing/Detoxifying: helps the body remove toxins and detoxifies the system and cleanses the digestive tract/colon.

Promotes Clarity: clears the mind and balances your mood.

Natural Weight Loss: burns excess fat, which stores harmful toxins.

Blast of Antioxidants: counteracts the free radicals that can cause cellular damage, aging, and susceptibility to cancers.

Natural Energy: no crashing or burning, but consistent energy.

Chlorophyll Rich: chlorophyll has a similar structure to hemoglobin that allows it to enhance the body's ability to produce more, which in turn enhances the delivery of oxygen to the cells; more oxygen to the cells allows the system to function properly.

Healthier Hair, Healthier Nails, and Clearer Skin: the minerals and vitamins in the fruits and vegetables provide a more youthful look.

Preventative Medicine: anticancer, anti-inflammatory, healing, and reverses chronic illness.

Better Sleep

Fulfil Daily Recommendations of Fruits & Vegetables

Juicing vs. Blending

I am often asked which is better: juices or smoothies. The answer is that both offer great benefits. I drink juices and smoothies, but I drink a lot more fresh juices than smoothies. The reason is juicing provides rapid nutrients to my cells in minutes without my body having to exert energy to breakdown and process it.

Juicing (Juices)

Juices are made by using a juicer (juice extractor or juice press). What the juicer does to your produce is extract the liquid nutrients by separating the fiber. By removing the fiber you free up your digestive system from having to work hard to break down the food to make the nutrients available for absorption. Your body does not need to exert any energy to process the juice. Without the fiber all the nutrients become instantly available to enter the bloodstream in minutes. Giving your body fuel to function optimally and nourishing your cells at a cellular level. Juicing offers way more vitamins, minerals, and phytonutrients than smoothies, because of the amount of produce needed to make a glass. Try blending 2 cucumbers, a bunch of kale, 3 apples, 1 lemon, and a piece of ginger. You probably won't be able to fit all that in your blender, nor will you enjoy drinking its chunky consistency or even finish it in a sitting. With juicing you can pack more servings of fruits and veggies into a single serving of juice than you can into a smoothie.

Blending (Smoothies)

Smoothies are made using a blender. Vitamix, Blendtec, and Nutribullet are popular blenders and are not juicers. Smoothies consist of all parts of fruits and vegetables including its fibers. Blending does break down the fibers, which makes it a lot easier to digest but energy is still required by the body to extract the nutrients. Since the fibers are intact this allows the nutrients to be slowly released in the bloodstream without any increase in blood sugar. It takes a few hours to obtain all the vitamins and minerals from a smoothie. The fibers also make smoothies more filling than a juice and it's quicker to make and clean up.

If you are deficient/low in minerals and vitamins, which is a large percentage of the population, then juicing is the way to go. It's much easier to drink a head of celery with apples than to eat them whole. Beginning your day with fresh juice will provide your body with instant vitamins, minerals, enzymes, phytochemicals, and more. Doing this daily provides your body with high doses of naturally derived nutrients that have many immune boosting benefits, some of which can protect the body against toxins and diseases. There's certainly nothing wrong with including both juicing and smoothies in your health regimen. For the purpose of this guide, we'll focus on juicing.

Why Drink Green Juices?

"Drinking just one freshly pressed juice each day is a reliable way of infusing your body with a wide variety of vitamins, minerals, and phytonutrients that can protect your cells against premature aging and disease." – Dr. Ben Kim

From what I know, green juicing was popularized through Ann Wigmore and Dr. Max Gerson. I'm not sure who brought it to the world first, but both used green juices and wheatgrass to heal themselves. Ann Wigmore healed herself from cancer more than 50 years ago. Her health center, Hippocrates Health Institute, has helped heal many people from chronic diseases and cancer by incorporating green juices, wheatgrass, and raw foods. The Gerson Therapy has done the same as well with cancer patients and people suffering from disease.

Green juice/vegetable juice benefits are numerous. Green juices and vegetable juices are very alkalizing, cleansing, healing, hydrating and restorative. Disease, inflammation, pain, and cancer all thrive in an acidic environment. You can rebuild muscle and damage cells through green juicing. Green juice offers a large cross-section of different nutrients from a variety of different greens and sprouts. Green juice supplies the body with chlorophyll. Chlorophyll has many benefits to the body; it neutralizes and removes toxins and heavy metals in the body, helps purify the liver, improves blood sugar problems, regulates digestion, helps rebuild tissues, antibacterial, and much more. A 32 oz. glass of fresh green juice may supply much of the protein an average adult needs each day. Believe it or not, leafy greens are 30% protein. Green vegetable juice won't spike your blood sugar and insulin level like an all fruit juice will. It's best to combine fruits in your green juices instead of drinking alone.

This is why I recommend a green juice a day. Health is wealth. All it takes is one glass of green juice. Do the best you can; start slow and enjoy the benefits

Getting Started

Selecting a Juicer

The first question any juice enthusiast asks is "what is the best juicer?" The simple answer is one that you will use consistently. The real answer is that there are various types of juicers on the market, priced from $40-$2000+. My motto is quality over quantity. That doesn't mean that the $2000+ juicer is the way to go. There are many options for beginners to elite juicers. I understand that a juicer is a serious investment. Below are many options depending on your price range and need.

Types of Juicers

Juicers can be broken down in to two main types: the centrifugal and masticating juicer.

Centrifugal Juicer

This is the most popular and affordable juicer on the current market. It's also readily available at local department stores worldwide. Centrifugal juicers work by spinning at a very high rpm (revolutions per minute, generally 13,000+ range), grating the fruits and vegetables into a pulp. The pulp gets expelled in the back chute and juice is released into the front glass.

Pros

- Fairly inexpensive, ranging from $40-$300

- Can process lots of whole fruits and vegetables in whole pieces. (Little chopping is required)
- Makes juice quickly
- Easy to clean and use (Takes max 15 minutes to setup, make juice, and clean up)

Cons
- Very loud
- The high speed of the spinning blade cause lots of oxygen to enter the juice. This causes the juice to oxidize destroying a portion of the enzymes and nutrients.
- Does not process leafy greens and grass well, very little juice is produced.
- Lots of wet pulp is produced, means not all juice is extracted, and equals wasted juice
- Short shelf-life, must consume immediately for most nutrition.
- Limited warranty about 1 year

So who is this style of juicer for?
Anyone looking for an affordable juicer and/or a juicer that doesn't take up much time

Some popular centrifugal juicers
- Breville
- Jack Lalane

Masticating Juicer

Masticating juicers are the most effective and efficient juicers, producing nutrient-dense juice. These juicers are more efficient because they can extract more juice from the same amount of produce used with a centrifugal juicer. Masticating juicers also run at a much slower rpm (average 80 rpm) than the centrifugal juicer. Masticating juicers can juice fruits, vegetables, leafy greens, and grasses extremely well.

There are two types of masticating juicers: the single auger and twin gear. The single auger is a single gear that chews/crushes and breaks down the fruit/vegetable fibers and cell walls. The twin gear juicers operate by crushing food through two interlocking gears. This style of juicer runs at a much slower speed than the single auger. Much more juice is produced, releasing more enzymes, nutrients, vitamins, and trace minerals.

Pros
- Quiet
- Efficiently juices fruits, vegetables, leafy greens, and grasses
- Produces much drier pulp, resulting in more juice, nutrients, vitamins and minerals
- Can store juice up to 3 days
- Runs at slow rpm, thus little to no foam produced and minimal oxidation
- Other functions, create nut butters, sorbets, pasta, and more
- Long warranty 10+ years (varies with brands)

Cons
- Pricey $230+
- Runs slower than centrifugal, thus requiring more time to make juice
- Heavier than centrifugal juicer

So who is this style of juicer for?

Those seeking highly mineralized juice, those wanting to rebuild their health, and those suffering from health challenges.

Some popular masticating juicers
- Omega 8006
- Omega Vert
- Super Angel Juicer 5500
- The Champion Juicer
- Norwalk (The best juicer on the market)

Please note: Be aware that to begin your green juice and juicing journey, you'll need the right juicer, one that will process both fruits and greens effectively. Invest in a good-quality juicer. Cheaper, centrifugal juicers introduce heat and oxygen and destroy some nutrients in your fruits and vegetables. My recommendation would be to select a masticating juicer. Masticating juicers are the best juicers for processing fruits, greens, and sprouts such as wheatgrass. I am currently using the omega 8005 juicer. Omega makes a great line of affordable masticating juicers.

Where to Buy Juicers

With the popularity of juicing, juicers are now more readily available in many major department stores. I picked up my Omega 8005 juicer off Amazon. Free shipping and no need to go anywhere. Amazon is available worldwide and carries a variety of centrifugal and masticating juicers. The one and only rule is to do the best you can with what you have. Any juicer you select within your budget and requirements will add beneficial nutrients to your body.

My top three recommendations for masticating juicers: Omega 8006 (8003, 8004. 8005, 8006 all similar), The Angel juicer, and The Norwalk

Tip 1. If the juicer cost is too high, grab a friend or two and spilt the cost. This will also be a great support system as you all begin your green juice journey.

Tip 2. Wash your juicer right after using to prevent the formation of bad bacteria, mildew, and other gross stuff. It's much easier to clean when you wash right away.

Tip 3. Keep your juicer on your counter or a viewable location. This will increase your usage. After all you've made an investment in your juicer; it's only best to use it often. I like to say get your monies worth ;-)

Other Equipment

Below are some useful additions to go along with your juicer.

- Vegetable Brush
    - To remove dirt from your vegetables and fruit skins
- Chopping Board
- Sharp Knife
- Peeler
- Mason Jars
    - I use mason jars to store and drink my juices. They are made out glass and free of plastic and harmful BPAs. Freezer safe. They also keep your juices airtight so that your juice will last longer and stay fresher, if you plan to consume later
- BPA Free Mason Jar Lid
    - These lids are plastic but BPA free. The metal lids that come with the mason jars will rust over time. You'll need to replace them often or you can go with these.
- Nut Milk Bag / Mesh Strainer
    - Strain your juice to remove any small bits or if you want a really smooth juice.

Selecting Produce

Organic Vs. Conventional Produce

Here's the deal with organic produce: rule #1 choose organic over conventional whenever possible. Here's why. To get the healthiest most nutrient dense juice possible, you'll want to buy organic. It's important because pesticides, fungicides, herbicides, and whatever-cides are heavily used on conventional produce. So what does this mean to us? In 1995 the USDA tested roughly 7,000 conventionally grown fruit and vegetable produce and found residue of 65 different types of pesticide, with 2 out of 3 samples containing pesticide residue. Pesticide residue has been shown to cause numerous long-term health risks, such as cancer and birth defects, nerve damage, impaired fertility, and more.

"Laboratory studies show that pesticides can cause health problems, such as birth defects, nerve damage, cancer, and other effects that might occur over a long period of time..." – EPA (US Environmental Protection Agency)

So by choosing organic produce over conventional, you are avoiding the harmful effects of pesticides, but you are also consuming higher quality foods that are higher in nutritional content. A 2001 study published in the Journal of Alternative and Complementary Medicine found that organic produce contained 27% more vitamin C, 21% more iron and 29% more magnesium than conventional produce and much more.

If money is an issue there are 12 produce you must buy organic. These are known as the dirty dozen. They are known as this because of the higher amounts of pesticides and other chemicals they contain.

Dirty Dozen

1. Apples

2. Celery

3. Strawberries

4. Peaches

5. Spinach

6. Nectarines (Imported)

7. Grapes (Imported)

8. Bell Peppers

9. Potatoes

10. Blueberries

11. Lettuce

12. Kale and Collard Greens

*These are the produce you should buy organic, because they contain the most pesticide residue. Everything else is fair game if money is an issue.

Tip. Don't over-buy produce. It is best to buy fresh produce every 3-4 days. This prevents spoilage. You can do this by planning out which recipes you'll juice for those days and calculating the amount of produce you will need.

Selecting Produce to Juice

Always select fresh produce both for juicing and eating. Fresh produce not only taste better, but contain higher quality nutrients. Avoid discolored vegetables and wilted leaves; opt for dark vibrant colors and crisp leaves. Avoid overripe fruits, because they will clog your juicers. Instead eat them or save for a smoothie. Select firm fruits for juicing.

How to Buy Affordable Organic Produce

I spend on average $25-$30 a week on organic fruits and vegetable and that's for myself and my partner. I used to easily spend double that if not more at places like Whole Foods aka Whole Paycheck. Following these tips that I am going to share with you will help keep more money in your pocket and allow you to get much more for less than what you used to pay for.

Support Local Farmers

The bulk of my fruits and vegetables come from my local farmers market. It's my favorite place to shop, because I get amazing deals and the fruits and veggies are so fresh. They are picked the day before, instead of weeks or even months before like in regular grocery stores. They don't come from other countries; many produce in grocery stores come from faraway place like Mexico, Asia, Canada, and South America.

Here are some tips while shopping at your local farmers market:

1. Prices are negotiable towards the end of the market.

2. If you shop there often, farmers will take care of you. Develop a relationship with your farmer. I'm a regular and I'm always given extra goods, 2 for the price of 1.

3. Buy in bulk. Discounts are given when you buy in bulk, anywhere from 20-30%. Apples, pears, carrots, beets, and other fruits can be stored longer than leafy greens. I don't eat all my berries, so I freeze them for later use.

4. Buy the ugly stuff often called seconds. I don't know about you, but I don't need a perfectly round apple. These fruits are often discount up to 50%. Seconds only means that the appearance is imperfect, but not the quality. If there is no sign, don't be afraid to ask.

The easiest way to find a local farmers market in your area is to Google search: [your city] [farmers market]

Join A CSA

A CSA, or community supported agriculture, is another way you can buy local and seasonal foods directly from a farmer. Each week you'll receive a box of fruits and vegetables and other farm products may be included. All depends on the package you decide to select. Essentially it's a weekly subscription of the freshest produce that is in season. It's a great way to try new vegetables for new ways of cooking.

To find a local CSA check out:

http://www.localharvest.org/csa/

http://www.biodynamics.com/csa.html

http://www.buylocalfood.com

Grow Your Own Foods

I like this option a lot. It's a great way to get outdoor exercise, sunshine (free vitamin D), and de-stress/relax. You can grow in your backyard and/or indoors. Even if you don't have space there are other options like joining a community garden. I have a hydroponic system set up to grow herbs and I also joined a local community garden in my neighborhood in the city of Chicago.

Membership Warehouse Clubs

Here's another option: you can become a member at Costco from $55/year. These warehouse stores allow for bulk buying at a discounted price. They contain a fair amount of organic produce that you can buy in addition to other household needs.

Dirty Dozen

If for some reason none of the above options are available to you, focus on purchasing these 12 fruits and vegetables organically. Every year for the past 8 years, the Environmental Working Group (EWG) collects data on foods contaminated with pesticides. These 12 fruits and vegetables are found to have the highest amount of pesticides, so it is crucial to buy them organic. [List is on page 12]

Fruit and Vegetable Prep for Juicing

Washing Your Produce

Before you juice your produce, it is best to thoroughly wash them. Bacteria and other germs get transferred between the dozens of people who come into contact with the produce. A simple cold water bath with the addition of 1 cup white vinegar or food grade hydrogen peroxide will do. You can also use a veggie wash or make your own with one part vinegar to three parts distilled water. Use a food brush to remove grit and dirt.

Use the Leaves and Stems

Include leaves and stems that come with your produce while juicing. They are loaded with nutrients. The only exception to this rule is carrot tops (or carrot greens). They contain compounds that may act as toxins in the bodies of certain individuals.

Remove Pits

To prevent any damage to your juicers, make sure to remove any hard pits from fruits you plan to juice. Fruits such as peaches, plums, nectarines, and apricots.

Remove the Outer Skins of Citrus Fruits

The skin of citrus fruits like grapefruits, oranges, tangerines etc. should not be juiced. The skins are extremely bitter and they contain oils that can cause digestive discomfort. Lemons and limes are the exception. You can juice them whole or remove the skins. When removing the skins of citrus fruits for juicing do make sure to keep as much of the white pith on. They are rich in vitamin C, quercetin, and other antioxidants.

Cut Fruits and Vegetables for Juicing

When you are ready to juice, cut your fruits and vegetables small enough to fit into the opening of your juicer to prevent any jamming or clogging.

Storing Your Produce

Proper storage of your produce is important, this helps minimize waste, spoilage, and money. You can store your produce right away in airlock bags or containers. The Evert-Fresh green bags allow your produce to stay fresher longer. If you're a busy person, I find it more effective to wash all produce, thoroughly dry them, and then place them in airlock bags. This saves time when juicing. All you'll have to do is grab your pre-washed produce and juice. Below is a method I use to help keep my leafy greens and herbs crisp and fresh until my next trip to the grocery store.

These steps will work for all lettuces, dark leafy greens (ex: kale and collards), and rough herbs (ex: parsley and dill).

1. Remove any rubber bands or elastic that is around the produce.

2. Create a cold bath in your kitchen sink. I like to add a ½ cup of vinegar. Veggie wash works just as well. This helps kill any harmful bacteria and gets rid of any other residue on your produce.

3. Soak for about 20-30 minutes. Swirl the produce around a few times. If there is heavy dirt on your greens or lettuce, use your fingers or a soft bristle brush to remove it.

4. To speed up the drying process, I use my trusty salad spinner. If you don't have a salad spinner, consider getting one, because it's a very useful kitchen gadget. Who wants to have wet salad leaves? Trust me; it will change your life.

* If you don't have a salad spinner, make sure to towel dry completely and lay out for about 15 minutes on a paper towel.

Please note that you can reuse these paper towels. I like to leave them out to dry and use for the next time.

Now that you've thoroughly washed and dried your produce, you must properly store them. **Proper storage is key to longer lasting fruits and vegetables.**

5. You can use ziploc containers, ziploc bags, store produce bags, or green bags (**ex:** Evert Fresh bags) to store your greens and herbs. Wrap your lettuce, greens, and herbs with paper towels. **The paper towels will absorb moisture, preventing leaves from turning limp and/or moldy.**

6. Place them into the bags or green bags and store in your refrigerator. If you are using a container, line the inside of your container with paper towels and place your greens inside. Place the lid on the container and refrigerate.

* Keep your greens closer to the front to prevent any freezing. If space is limited make sure the stems or tips are pointed towards the back, just in case any freezing occurs. You can just cut of the stems should that occur.

The benefit of following this procedure is that once you've washed and stored your produce for the week, it's ready to use. It cuts the time down tremendously. All it takes is about 30 minutes once week or twice a week, depending on however many times you head to the grocery store or market.

Your leafy greens and herbs will keep up to a week; some will even keep up to two weeks.

*Special tip: if you've brought back semi-wilted greens, you can soak them in cold water for 30 minutes or overnight. This method will help revive your greens.

Storing Your Juices

To get the maximum nutrition from your juices, it is best to consume them once they are made, within twenty minutes. This is because the nutritional value will decline once exposed to air/oxygen. In a perfect world this would be possible, but not everyone can do this, ex. work. With proper storage you can still get an excellent source of nutrition from your juices.

The best storage for your fresh juices are glass mason jars or stainless steel jars. They contain no chemicals or toxins (BPA) that can leech into your drink like that of a plastic bottle. The key to preventing nutrient loss in stored juices is to make sure you fill your juice to the top of the jar, so that there is no oxygen in the bottle. Keep your juices in a cool and dark environment. Store them in a cooler if you plan to take with you. It's also important to note that juice from a masticating juicer will remain fresher longer than juice from a high speed centrifugal juicer. Juices from a masticating juicer can be refrigerated for 3-5 days. Juices from centrifugal juicers can be refrigerated for 24-48 hours. If you need to store longer, freezing is another option. If you are planning to freeze your juice, do it right after it is made.

Proper Juicing Etiquette

It is best to drink your juice on an empty stomach. Drinking your juices along with food or a full stomach can cause fermentation (gas) and other stomach discomforts. It also slows down nutrient absorption. If you plan on having a meal, it best to drink your juices thirty minutes before your meal or an hour or more after your meal.

Sip your juices; don't chug them. Sipping your juice also allows your body to properly assimilate each nutrient.

Cleaning Your Juicer

This is probably the least exciting part about juicing. Once you are finished juicing it is best to clean/wash your juicer right away. It is much easier and faster to clean a juicer that you just used than a juicer that has been sitting in the sink. Leaving your dirty juicer for later causes the pulpy remains to harden and also creates a breeding nest for fruit flies and other critters. It will only take you 60 seconds to clean, so do it right away.

Now that you know everything there is to get started juicing, lets dive into the 7 day plan.

7 Day Juice Plan

Let's get started. I've provided a juice recipe for each day of the week. There's no need to change anything drastic in your current diet, but if you're eating poorly consider also adding in some fresh fruits and vegetables in addition to your daily juice. Each recipe will make about 16-20oz of juice. This is one serving. If you want more juice, by all means double the recipe. If you're new to juicing, use this first week as an introduction. You'll want to allow your body to make the necessary adjustments. You can consume these juices at any time of the day, but I recommend starting your day with a fresh glass of green juice. After you've done that you can proceed with your daily meal.

Monday – Sweet Cucumber

4 Handfuls of Spinach (Swiss chard is another great substitute)
2 Cucumbers
2 Medium Fuji Apples

Spinach is among the top healthiest vegetables, loaded with a full spectrum of vitamins and minerals along with anti-inflammatory and anti-cancer properties.
The health benefits of spinach include: anticancer, improves mental function, heart protector, antioxidant, anti-cataracts, and anti-anemia.

Nutrition Information

1 Serving (16-20 oz.)

Calories 268.9

Total Carbohydrate 63.2 g

Total Fat 1.7 g

Sodium 106.8 mg

Potassium 1,854.1 mg

Protein 8.0 g

Sugar 24g

Vitamin A: 253.7 %

Vitamin B-6: 31.0 %

Vitamin C: 135.6 %

Vitamin E: 18.0 %

Calcium: 22.3 %

Copper: 23.5 %

Folate: 79.8 %

Iron: 29.6 %

Magnesium: 43.9 %

Manganese: 82.9 %

Niacin: 12.2 %

Pantothenic Acid: 13.3 %

Phosphorus: 19.9 %

Riboflavin: 23.4 %

Selenium: 2.9 %

Thiamin: 19.0 %

Zinc: 12.9 %

*Percent Daily Values are based on a 2,000 calorie diet. Your daily values may be higher or lower depending on your calorie needs.

Tuesday – Mighty Green

3 Celery Ribs
1 ½ Cucumber
½ Parsley Bunch
1 Apple

Parsley is an excellent source of vitamin C and vitamin A (beta-carotene). These two nutrients have been linked to reduced risks of heart disease, colon cancer, diabetes, asthma, and arthritis. Parsley helps the body get rid of excess water and flush the kidneys.

Nutrition Information
1 Serving (16-20 oz.)
Calories 214.1

Total Fat 2.0 g
Total Carbohydrate 48.2 g
Sugars 14.8 g
Protein 8.3 g
Sodium 243.3 mg
Potassium 2,024.8 mg

Vitamin A 228.1 %
Vitamin B-6 26.5 %
Vitamin C 341.4 %
Vitamin E 18.1 %
Calcium 31.6 %
Copper 22.6 %
Folate 74.7 %
Iron 53.5 %
Magnesium 34.5 %
Manganese 39.7 %

Niacin 16.6 %
Pantothenic Acid 17.3 %
Phosphorus 21.8 %
Riboflavin 19.0 %
Selenium 3.2 %
Thiamin 21.6 %
Zinc 16.5 %

*Percent Daily Values are based on a 2,000 calorie diet. Your daily values may be higher or lower depending on your calorie needs.

Wednesday – Kale Pineapple Mint

1 Cucumber
1 Granny Smith Apple
1 Cup Pineapple
3 Kale Leaves
1 Handful Mint
½ Lemon (remove peel)

Kale is one of the most nutrient dense foods. Some of its health benefits include immune boosting, cardiovascular support, skin-healing, bone-building, and aids in detoxification. They are also loaded with anti-cancer nutrients. Kale nutritional properties have been shown to lower your risk of at least five different types of cancer, which include cancer of the bladder, breast, colon, ovary, and prostate. There are at least 4 different kale varieties sold in grocery stores, including all varieties in your diet.

Nutrition Information

1 Serving (16-20 oz.)

Calories 273.6

Total Fat 2.5 g

Total Carbohydrate 67.8 g

Sodium 66.9 mg

Potassium 1,445.2 mg

Sugars 29.8 g

Protein 7.9 g

Vitamin A 427.6 %

Vitamin B-6 37.3 %

Vitamin C 416.9 %

Vitamin E 4.2 %

Calcium 27.7 %

Copper 43.5 %

Folate 25.2 %

Iron 23.1 %

Magnesium 29.1 %

Manganese 194.5 %

Niacin 13.8 %

Pantothenic Acid 12.0 %

Phosphorus 16.9 %

Riboflavin 19.6 %

Selenium 3.9 %

Thiamin 27.7 %

Zinc 9.5 %

*Percent Daily Values are based on a 2,000 calorie diet. Your daily values may be higher or lower depending on your calorie needs.

Thursday – Green Peace

5 Kale Leaves
1 Cucumber
½ Lemon
2 Fuji Apples

Cucumber's high water content and mineral balance hydrates your body down to the cellular level. Cucumbers top three phytonutrients are cucurbitacins, lignans, and flavonoids. These specific phytonutrients provide our bodies with antioxidant, anti-inflammatory, and anti-cancer benefits. In addition, cucumbers nourish the skin, cleanse the kidneys, and help reduce cholesterol.

Nutrition Information

1 Serving (16-20 oz.)

Calories 311.9

Total Fat 2.5 g

Total Carbohydrate 76.4 g

Sodium 94.0 mg

Potassium 1,726.3 mg

Sugars 27.6 g

Protein 9.7 g

Vitamin A 634.1 %

Vitamin B-6 42.9 %

Vitamin C 524.1 %

Vitamin E 5.6 %

Calcium 36.5 %

Copper 47.8 %

Folate 26.8 %

Iron 27.3 %

Magnesium 31.5 %

Manganese 95.6 %

Niacin 14.1 %

Pantothenic Acid 11.4 %

Phosphorus 20.8 %

Riboflavin 22.4 %

Selenium 4.2 %

Thiamin 24.7 %

Zinc 11.0 %

*Percent Daily Values are based on a 2,000 calorie diet. Your daily values may be higher or lower depending on your calorie needs.

Friday – Incredible Hulk

2 Cucumbers
2 Pears
½ Lemon
½ in Ginger root (size should be the equivalent to tip of your thumb)
½ Kale Bunch

Next to apples, pears are fruits that can be used in any juice recipe. They help protect the colon and contain antioxidant and anti-inflammatory properties.

Lemons and all citrus fruits contain compounds (lycopene and limonene) that can fight against cancer.

Nutrition Information

1 Serving (16-20 oz.)

Calories 352.6

Total Fat 2.9 g

Total Carbohydrate 85.5 g

Sodium 100.6 mg

Potassium 2,275.5 mg

Sugars 27.4 g

Protein 12.5 g

Vitamin A 645.6 %

Vitamin B-6 45.9 %

Vitamin C 547.0 %

Vitamin E 10.7 %

Calcium 42.4 %

Copper 66.2 %

Folate 40.5 %

Iron 33.6 %

Magnesium 41.7 %

Manganese 114.0 %

Niacin 18.0 %

Pantothenic Acid 17.5 %

Phosphorus 28.6 %

Riboflavin 32.0 %

Selenium 7.9 %

Thiamin 30.9 %

Zinc 17.1 %

*Percent Daily Values are based on a 2,000 calorie diet. Your daily values may be higher or lower depending on your calorie needs.

Saturday – Mr. Clean

4 Kale Leaves
3 Celery Ribs
1 Cucumber
½ in Ginger root
½ Lemon
2 Apples (Fuji/Gala)

Apples are an excellent addition to any juice recipe. Not only do they make a great base for your juices, they contain many health properties from vitamins, minerals, and malic acid for cleansing and detoxification benefits, digestion aid, cholesterol lowering, and improved condition of the skin. There are many varieties of apples to try. Some of my favorite are fujis, galas, and pink lady apples. Red Delicious tend to have a lot more sugar, whereas the Granny Smith variety is one that has lower sugar content

Nutrition Information

1 Serving (16-20 oz.)

Calories 301.7

Total Fat 2.2 g

Total Carbohydrate 74.8 g

Sodium 170.2 mg

Potassium 1,790.0 mg

Sugars 27.7 g

Protein 8.5 g

Vitamin A 431.3 %

Vitamin B-6 39.5 %

Vitamin C 404.5 %

Vitamin E 7.8 %

Calcium 32.4 %

Copper 40.3 %

Folate 30.3 %

Iron 24.1 %

Magnesium 29.3 %

Manganese 76.3 %

Niacin 13.2 %

Pantothenic Acid 12.7 %

Phosphorus 20.0 %

Riboflavin 20.7 %

Selenium 4.8 %

Thiamin 23.5 %

Zinc 10.1

*Percent Daily Values are based on a 2,000 calorie diet. Your daily values may be higher or lower depending on your calorie needs.

Sunday – Green Detox

1 Cucumber
3 Granny Smith Apples
4 Kale Leaves
3 Swiss Chard Leaves
5 Sprigs of Parsley
1 Celery Rib

Swiss chard, like many leafy greens, offers a rich source of chlorophyll that can alkalize the body. Over acidic bodies cater to disease and disharmony. Swiss chard is packed with nutrients that support bone health and help regulate blood sugar. Like many leafy greens, swiss chard offers anticancer, antioxidant, and anti-inflammatory benefits.

Nutrition Information

1 Serving (16-20 oz.)

Calories 392.8

Total Fat 2.2 g

Total Carbohydrate 94.0 g

Sodium 414.5 mg

Potassium 2,611.1 mg

Sugars 43.4 g

Protein 10.8 g

Vitamin A 653.0 %

Vitamin B-6 43.7 %

Vitamin C 402.1 %

Vitamin E 25.4 %

Calcium 37.7 %

Copper 49.0 %

Folate 31.4 %

Iron 45.1 %

Magnesium 65.0 %

Manganese 104.4 %

Niacin 15.3 %

Pantothenic Acid 13.8 %

Phosphorus 24.1 %

Riboflavin 27.5 %

Selenium 6.6 %

Thiamin 25.0 %

Zinc 13.5 %

*Percent Daily Values are based on a 2,000 calorie diet. Your daily values may be higher or lower depending on your calorie needs.

Shopping List

9 Cucumbers

1 Spinach Bunch or 1-5oz Bag

10 Fuji Apples (Gala or Braeburn or Honeycrisp or Jonagold)

1 Head of Celery

4 Granny Smith Apples

1 Parsley Bunch

1 Pineapple

2 Kale Bunches

1 Mint Bunch or 1-2oz Container

2 Lemons

2 Pears

Ginger Root (No more than 3 inch long)

1 Swiss Chard Bunch

How to Make Green Juice Template

Making green juice is very easy. Below is a basic formula you can follow to create various combinations.

1. Select your base (1 or more)

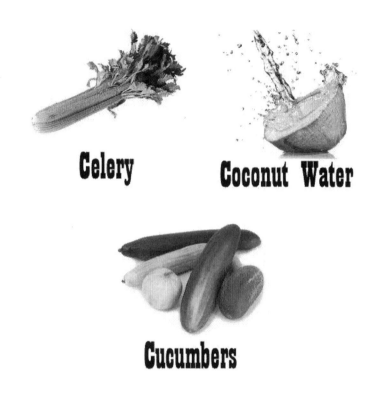

Celery

Coconut Water

Cucumbers

The base makes up the bulk of your juice. You can select one or two or all three.

2. Select your leafy greens (Add 1 or more variety)

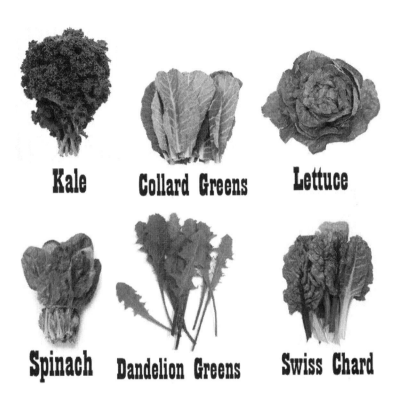

Start with 2 handfuls per juice.

3. Add Herbs (add 1 or 2 herbs)

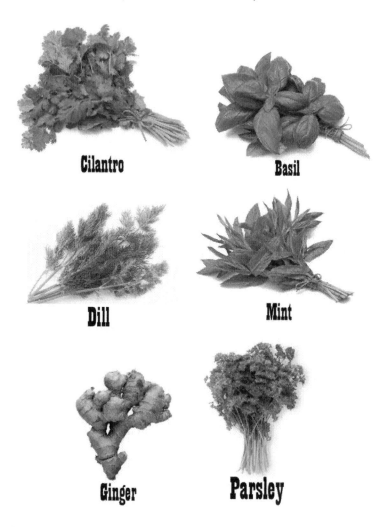

Cilantro

Basil

Dill

Mint

Ginger

Parsley

Start with a handful per juice. For the ginger root, start with a 1/2in piece, about the size of the tip of your thumb.

4. Sweeten up (1 or more)

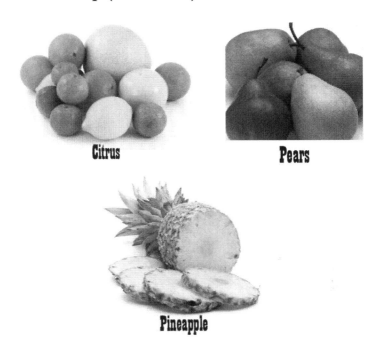

Citrus

Pears

Pineapple

4. Sweeten up (1 or more) - continued

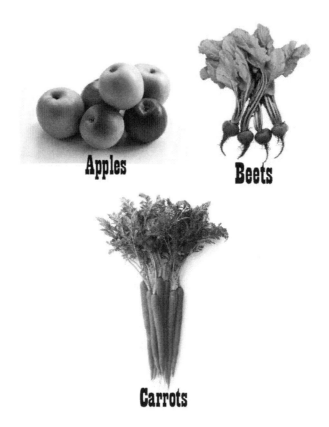

Apples

Beets

Carrots

The amount is up to you. If you want sweeter use more.

5. Add sprouts (Optional) (Use if available, sprouts are 10-30x more nutritious than the best vegetable.)

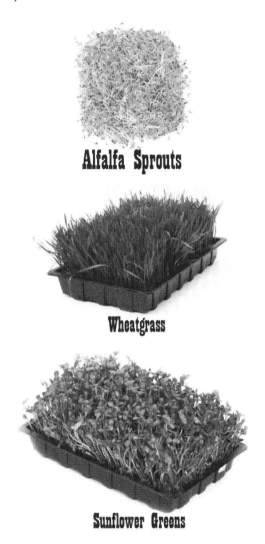

Alfalfa Sprouts

Wheatgrass

Sunflower Greens

*If adding wheatgrass, begin with 1 oz of liquid first a day. Wheatgrass is very potent and cleansing. Select other mild sprouts if you are a beginner.

6. Add-ons (Optional)

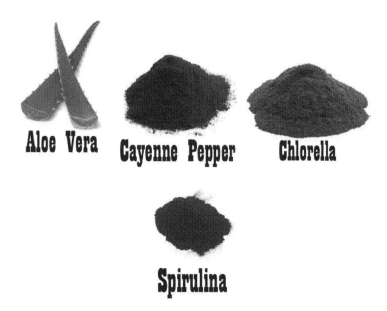

Aloe Vera   **Cayenne Pepper**   **Chlorella**

Spirulina

A pinch of cayenne pepper goes a long way.

7. Juice all 5 components

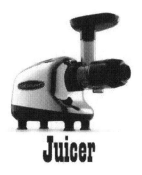

Juicer

Fruit and Vegetable Flavor Families

Fruits and vegetables all have different types of flavors. Below you'll find the flavor groupings of fruits and vegetables. You can apply this chart for future juicing experiments, substitutions, and/or with meal recipes.

Fruit: Tart
Papayas, blueberries, kumquats, quinces, grapes, cherries, pineapple, kiwis
Fruit: Sweet
Watermelon, clementines, peaches, navel oranges, dates, figs, nectarines, mangoes, honeydew melon
Fruit: Mild
Apricots, strawberries, bananas, cantaloupe, pears, pluots, plums
Fruit: Crisp
Honeydew melon, Asian pears, summer apples, pears
Fruit: Smooth
Mangoes, bananas, dates, figs, apricots
Vegetables: Grassy
Celery, asparagus, chard, spinach, mizuna, cucumbers, green beans
Vegetables: Sweet
Bell peppers, snap peas, beets, carrots, fennel, sweet potatoes, parsnips
Vegetables: Spicy

Radishes, onions, turnips, watercress, arugula, leeks, chile peppers, basil	
Vegetables: Bitter	
Chicory, radicchio, frisee, dandelion leaves, eggplant, escarole	
Vegetables: Earthy	
Beets, broccoli, cabbage, collards, kohlrabi, chard, mushrooms, rutabagas	
Vegetables: Neutral	
Zucchini, chard, iceberg lettuce, daikon, eggplant, potatoes, spinach	
Vegetables: Tart	
Lemongrass, sorrel, tomatillos	
Vegetables: Buttery	
Artichokes, peas, edamame, mushrooms, asparagus, avocados	
Vegetables: Anise	
Fennel, basil, endive	

(Source: http://www.wholeliving.com/136106/fruit-and-vegetable-flavor-families)

* Bananas, avocados, mushrooms, artichokes, dates, and potatoes (sweet potatoes are okay) are not suitable for juicing.

Vegetable & Fruit Substitution List

Depending on your location, some of the vegetables and fruits in the recipes may not be available. Below is an excellent substitution list. This list isn't for juicing alone. You can use it for preparing meals as well.

Items	Substitutions
Apple	Any variety, pear, red grapes, black grapes, cherries, blackberries, blueberries
Arugula (Rocket)	Spinach, kale, watercress
Avocado	Roasted veggies (squash, mushroom, eggplant), banana, olive
Banana	Avocado
Basil	Parsley, cilantro, mint
Beets (Beetroot)	Golden beets, red cabbage, tomato, radish
Blueberries	Blackberries, strawberries, raspberries, cherries
Bok Choy	Kale, beet greens, dandelion greens
Broccoli stalk	Celery, cucumber, cauliflower
Broccoli	Cauliflower, green cabbage
Butternut squash	Pumpkin, carrot, sweet potato, acorn squash, spaghetti squash, delicata squash, Hubbard squash
Cantaloupe (Rockmelon)	Mango, papaya, peach
Carrots	Sweet potato/yam, winter squash, pumpkin, parsnip
Celeriac root	Celery, turnip, parsley root, kohlrabi, jicama, daikon

Celery	Cucumber, zucchini, jicama
Cherries	Raspberries, strawberries, blackberries
Chives	Scallion
Cilantro (Coriander)	Basil, parsley
Coconut water	Water, diluted fresh juice
Collard Greens	Mustard greens, kale, beet greens, dandelion greens
Cranberries	Cherries, raspberries
Cucumber	Celery, zucchini, jicama
Dandelion Greens	Kale, mustard or collard greens, beet greens
Eggplant	Mushrooms
Fennel	Celeriac root, kohlrabi, jicama, daikon, endive
Garlic	Shallot
Ginger	Lemon
Grapefruit	Another variety of grapefruit, clementine, orange, tangerine, blood orange, star fruit
Green Beans	Asparagus, long bean, French bean
Green cabbage	Red/purple cabbage, kale, arugula, watercress, endive
Green peppers (Capsicum)	Red or yellow peppers, mushrooms
Honeydew (Melon)	Green grapes, avocado
Jalapeno (Chili pepper)	Serrano pepper, yellow wax pepper, chile pepper of choice
Kale (Tuscan cabbage)	Arugula, watercress, spinach, Swiss chard, green cabbage, mustard/collard/beet/turnip greens
Kiwifruit	Mango, orange, tangerine, lime
Lemon	Ginger

Lime	Lemon, orange, clementine/tangerine
Mango	Papaya, kiwifruit
Maple Syrup	Honey
Mint	Ginger, sweet basil
Onion	Garlic, leeks, shallot
Orange	Grapefruit, clementine, tangerine, kiwifruit, mango, papaya
Oregano	Sage
Parsley	Cilantro, kale, arugula
Parsnips	Turnip, parsley root, celeriac root
Peaches	Nectarines, plums
Pear	Apple, celery root, peach, plum
Pineapple	Orange, grapefruit, mango
Pomegranate	Pineapple, strawberries
Portobello Mushroom	Any variety mushroom, eggplant
Radish	Red cabbage, tomato
Raisins	Dried cranberries, figs
Red/purple cabbage	Green cabbage, radish, cauliflower, broccoli, radicchio
Romaine	Bib lettuce, radicchio, endive, Boston lettuce, green or red leaf lettuce
Shallot (Eschalot)	Garlic, onion
Spinach	Kale, Swiss chard, romaine lettuce
Strawberries	Raspberries, blackberries, cherries
Summer Squash	Zucchini, cucumber
Swiss Chard (Silverbeet)	Kale, spinach, romaine, mustard/collard/beet/turnip greens, green cabbage, arugula, watercress
Tangerines	Orange, grapefruit
Thyme	Rosemary
Tomato	Radish, red pepper, watermelon

Watermelon	Red grapefruit, cantaloupe, honeydew, tomato, radish
White Wine vinegar	Red wine vinegar, cider or champagne vinegar

Source: Reboot Holdings Pty. Ltd.

Frequently Asked Questions

What greens are easiest to juice?

For beginners it's best to start with spinach, swiss chard, and lettuce. You can find a variety of lettuces in the supermarket and/or farmers market. Some varieties are romaine, red leaf, green leaf, cos, boston, etc. Avoid iceberg lettuce. They lack nutrients.

What can I add to sweeten my juices?

Many options are available: apples, pears, citrus, pineapples, carrots, plums, berries kiwi, lemon, limes, stevia, and more. When you are first starting out, feel free to add as many apples and pears to make it suitable to your taste. Over time your taste buds will adjust and you'll find that you won't need to add a lot fruits. Diabetics should stick to low glycemic fruits like apples and pears to sweeten their juices.

How fast or slow can I consume my juice?

A general rule when you make your juice: it's best to drink it right away; when exposed to light and oxygen nutrients begin to oxidize. If you are not drinking it right away store it in an airtight mason jar for later consumption.

Can I refrigerate and how long?

You can refrigerate your juices. Just place them in an airtight mason jar and fill to the top. Juices made with a masticating juicer can last for 3-5 days. If made with centrifugal juicers drink within 24-48 hours.

Why is juicing better than store bought juice?

Store bought juices like Naked and Odwalla are owned by Coca Cola and Pepsi. They don't know anything about health. But really these juices are pasteurized, heated to the point where all the minerals, vitamins, and nutrients are gone. They are loaded questionable ingredients and they are very high in sugar. Drinking those juices will cause your blood sugar to spike and then will be followed with a crash. Fresh juices provide natural energy, vitamins, minerals, living enzymes, nutrients, and more.

What are the best juice combos?

Keep it simple. Start with a base of celery and/or cucumber or coconut water. Select one type of leafy greens and sweeten with fruit. An example: cucumbers, apples, and parsley. Very easy and refreshing.

Is juicing enough or should I eat something with it?

Depends on your body. If you find that you are hungry after drinking your juice, feel free to add a light meal after. You can combine your fresh juice with fruits or a large vegetable salad. Drink your juice first and follow it with food twenty minutes after.

What juice do you suggest for those with diabetes?

Green juices are perfect for diabetics. You can drink pure vegetable juices or you can sweeten with low glycemic fruits like green apples, green pears, limes, and lemons. Stevia is also a great addition for diabetics. Make sure to consult your doctor beforehand.

Can I prepare produce beforehand?

A great way to cut your juicing time down is prepare your produce beforehand. The night before, make sure all your produce is thoroughly washed and dried. Store what you plan to juice in a large BPA free container or Ziploc bag. It's best to chop fruits right before juicing because this keeps the nutrients intact. However, if you need to cut your fruits beforehand in order for you to juice, by all means do so. It's better to juice then to not juice at all. Rub fresh lemon on the fruits you plan to cut, lemon is a natural preserver.

What can I do with leftover pulp?

There are many ways you can use leftover pulp. You can create delicious flax crackers, muffins, and cakes, especially with carrot pulp. Additionally you can compost your pulp. You can add you pulp to soups as a thickening agent. You can add it to homemade burgers, veggie burgers, meat loaf, and/or nut loafs. For fruit pulps, they are great additions to oatmeal, muffins, or pancake mixes.

Can I juice with frozen fruits and vegetables?

Frozen vegetables are best for smoothies; however, if those are your only options, you can thaw them out and then juice. Most of the nutrients are still present in frozen fruits/vegetables.

My organic options are limited. What can I do to minimize pesticides and chemicals?

Make sure you thoroughly wash and scrub your fruits and vegetables. Use a veggie wash or add in a ¼ - ½ cup of white vinegar (or food grade hydrogen peroxide) to your water bath for soaking. Make sure you peel the skin, many conventional foods

How much juice should I drink?

It's always important to note, when introducing something new to your current diet, start off slowly. This will give your body time to adjust and acclimate itself. So if you're new to juicing start with 16oz each day.

Conclusion

Congratulations for successfully completing the 7 day quick start to green juicing. So what's next? Feel free to complete the plan again. Remember you can switch up the ingredients. Use the How to Make a Green Juice as a guide as well as the substitution list. Rotate your greens to get in each unique health benefits from the vegetables of your choosing and so you don't get bored with them. Don't worry about being perfect. If you worry too much, then you'll never get started. Always do the best you can with what is available to you. You can always make improvements along the way. Remember the road to optimal health isn't an overnight process. All you have to do is start and stay consistent.

I sincerely hope you enjoyed this book. If you have any questions feel free to shoot me an email over at http://www.greenjuiceaday.com or post on my **Facebook page**: Facebook.com/GreenJuiceADay

If you found this book useful please take a few seconds and leave an Amazon review here:
http://amzn.to/11gRqOK

It is most greatly appreciated. Thank you.

Don't forget your **Free Bonus** for purchasing this book exclusively to Kindle Customers →
http://www.greenjuiceaday.com/kindle-bonus

Notes